Factors Related to Aggressive Behaviors in Adolescents with Autism Spectrum Disorder

Factors Related to Aggressive Behaviors in Adolescents with Autism Spectrum Disorder

Sydney McGee

Copyright © 2021 by Sydney McGee.

ISBN:	Softcover	978-1-6698-0150-4
	eBook	978-1-6698-0159-7

All rights reserved. No part of this book may be reproduced or transmitted in any form or by any means, electronic or mechanical, including photocopying, recording, or by any information storage and retrieval system, without permission in writing from the copyright owner.

Any people depicted in stock imagery provided by Getty Images are models, and such images are being used for illustrative purposes only.
Certain stock imagery © Getty Images.

Print information available on the last page.

Rev. date: 11/26/2021

To order additional copies of this book, contact:
Xlibris
844-714-8691
www.Xlibris.com
Orders@Xlibris.com
834767

CONTENTS

Personal Experience ix

Chapter 1   Introduction 1
    Statement of the Problem 1
    Scope of the Problem 2
    Importance of the Research 3

Chapter 2   Literature Review 4
    Signs and Symptoms of ASD 4
    Background of ASD 5
    Applied Behavior Analysis (ABA) 6
    Risk Factors of Aggression among Adolescents with ASD 7
    Teaching Strategies 7
    Behavioral Strategies 8
    Triggers of Aggression 8
    Outcomes of Aggression with ASD 9
    Genetics in Adolescence with ASD 10
    Abuse and Neglect in Adolescence with ASD 11
    Quality of Life in ASD 11

Chapter 3   Theoretical Framework 13
    Operant Conditioning 13
    Positive reinforcement 14
    Negative reinforcement 14

Chapter 4   Addressing the Problem 16

Chapter 5   Conclusion 19
    Social Work Implication 19
    What is Theoretical Orientation? 21

  Experience of Theoretical Orientation..................................21
  Discourses shaped Theoretical Orientation.........................22
  Integrated new Perspectives 22
  Diversity and Inclusion 23
  Leadership Style 24
  Social Change...24
  Mindfulness of ASD...25
  Community Advocate 26

My Own Boss 29
Jewell's of Autism L.L.C...31
Reference..37

Factors Related to Aggressive Behaviors in Adolescents with Autism Spectrum Disorder

Acceptable- We all must accept who we are as individuals, everyone has a basic human right, and it is vital to accept and understand the nature of autism.

Unifying- We are a unit, together we must be supportive towards another, and help raise autism awareness.

Teaching-We must educate another about the importance of diversity. Everyone is gifted to be their unique way.

Individual-every individual deserves to be cherished, loved, and respected no matter the circumstances. Individuals with autism are the source of success because they have so much to offer in the world.

Success- We are inspirational leaders in our nation and will ensure students of autism will reach their fullest potential of success. Failure is not an option.

Meaning- Many people do not know the meaning of autism. Please take the time to research, write, sing, act, draw, dance, so you can understand the purpose of autism. Be Creative!

Note: *You can only learn how to love others until you love yourself. Be grateful for what you have and who you are. Never underestimate others because you do not know what they may be experiencing. I believe everyone is here on earth for a reason, individuals with autism have a purposeful meaning in life.*

Personal Experience

Over the years, my personal experience working with special needs has been a true gift. One of the highlights of my life is I have gotten to learn how to deal with all levels of ups and downs. Going through these difficult experiences taught me about the importance of patience, empathy, compassion, and openness. Individuals with autism have their unique direct wants and needs in life. It is vital to understand the challenges that come along with having ASD. Therefore, autistic individuals have their own stories and obstacles in their everyday lives. People with autism are indeed creative, unique, and different. I view people with autism as "superheroes" because the profession educates us to become loving and caring together as a community. It has been an amazing journey to work with individuals with autism spectrum disorder (ASD). The world can often become confusing and overwhelming, and it is essential to empower autistic people to face their traumatic experiences.

Note: Step out of your comfort zone and focus on helping people who are different than you. Help them cope with their trauma such as reading, writing, drawing, shopping, or other physical activities that are calm and enjoyable.

Chapter One

Introduction

According to Kanne & Mazurek (2011), autism spectrum disorder (ASD) is a lifelong neurodevelopmental disorder that presents a range of complex developmental disorders characterized by difficulties in social engagement and verbal and nonverbal communication. Kanne & Mazurek (2011) acknowledges how aggressive behavior has become a significant problem among adolescents with autism spectrum disorder (ASD). This research proposal will investigate the triggers of aggressive behaviors towards themselves and others (Kanne & Mazurek, 2011). The first chapter will be acknowledging the adverse outcomes of aggressive behaviors in adolescents with autism spectrum disorder (ASD) (Simó-Pinatella et al., 2019). In this chapter, there will be three sections presented: statement of the problem, the scope of the problem, and why this is an important research topic. The primary goal of this study is to evaluate the factors of aggressive behaviors in autism spectrum disorder (ASD) (Simó-Pinatella et al., 2019).

Statement of the Problem

Aggression has become a significant issue for caregivers, parents, and teachers of adolescents on the autism spectrum (Hanley et al., 2014). An attack can significantly affect a person's learning ability, preventing them from learning in a school setting (Hanley et al., 2014). When an adolescent with autism spectrum disorder (ASD) becomes physically aggressive towards their peers, there is a need for a more restrictive learning environment (Hanley et al., 2014). Instead of adolescents attending public school because of their aggressive behavior. A should address their developmental needs through intensive behavioral intervention services such as in-home services (Hanley et al., 2014). Furthermore, being afraid of aggressive incidents may increase their sense of isolation and decrease their quality of life. The focal point is to determine what factors are associated with aggressive behavior in adolescents with autism spectrum disorder (ASD) (Hanley et al., 2014).

Scope of the Problem

According to the Centers for Disease Control and Prevention (CDC) (2013), there are many adolescences affected by autism who benefit from other interventions such as social skills and interests. Approximately 1 in 5 students who suffer from abnormal behaviors will be diagnosed with autism spectrum disorder (ASD). Typically, the ages occur between 1 and 3 who develop challenging behaviors early (Centers Disease Control and Prevention, 2013). There is an estimate of 1 in 54 students diagnosed with autism spectrum disorder (ASD). Not to mention, 1 in 34 males identified with autism spectrum disorder (ASD) in the United States. Boys are four times more likely to be diagnosed with autism than girls (Centers Disease Control and Prevention, 2013). However, 1 in 144 females is diagnosed with autism spectrum disorder (ASD). It is reported that 20% to 30 % of Whites have a higher probability of developing autism spectrum disorder (ASD) than Blacks. Besides, at least 70% of students have an average proportion of intellectual ability (Centers Disease Control and Prevention, 2013).

Importance of the Research

It is essential to understand why adolescence with autism are behaving aggressively and what they are trying to communicate (Escorcia, 2018). In addition, Escorcia (2018) utilizes methods to teach youth how to manage their aggressive outbursts. Therefore, the purpose of this research paper is to focus on improving the assessment and treatment of aggressive behavior and an evaluation of the individual exhibiting aggressive behaviors (Brentani et al., 2013). An assessment can tell the person why behaviors occur and implement strategies to help reduce abnormal behaviors (Brentani et al., 2013).

The ultimate goal is to control abnormal behaviors of autism and the impact it has on the individual, families, and the environment (Sullivan et al., 2019). Furthermore, the study of aggressive behavior is critical because helping autistic individuals will teach them to: learn how to control their anger, express anger and frustrations properly, it will also lead the individual how to be held responsible for their actions and accept the consequences (Sullivan et al., 2019). Also, family conflicts, school problems, and community issues are factors to address the causes of abnormal behavior in autism spectrum disorder (ASD) (Sullivan et al., 2019).

Chapter Two

Literature Review

To better understand the aggressive behaviors of adolescents with ASD, will be discussed in eleven sections; will discuss the aggressive behaviors of adolescents with ASD, the factors of autism will discuss the literature review in eleven areas; a) signs and symptoms, b) background of (ASD), c) applied behavior analysis (ABA), d) risk factors of aggression among adolescent with (ASD), e) teaching strategies, f) behavioral strategies, g) triggers of aggression, h) outcomes of aggression, i) genetics in (ASD), j) abuse, k) neglect and l) quality of life in (ASD). Aggressive behaviors can be challenging and frustrating for autistic adolescents to control their maladaptive behaviors. It is essential to understand that aggressive behaviors are tougher to overcome. The purpose of this study is to address aggressive behaviors in adolescents so they can live productive lives. Chapter two will focus on several factors related to aggressive behaviors in adolescents with autism spectrum disorder (ASD).

Signs and Symptoms of ASD

There are signs and symptoms of autism spectrum disorder (ASD): difficulty communicating and interacting with others, preference to their routine, dislike of change, anxiety, depression, and lack of interest in peer relationships (May et al., 2012). Adolescent who develops autism cannot express themselves or the disturbing situations that trigger them to react aggressively (Escorcia, 2018). For example, if autistic adolescents have trouble with their teeth or abdominal pain, they may not explain their situation, so their reaction will be aggressive (Escorcia, 2018). Kanne & Mazurek (2011) indicates how aggression and temper tantrums can be challenging for parents, which leads the child to develop repetitive behaviors.

Background of ASD

Kanne & Mazurek (2011) estimated how often aggressive behavior occurs in children and adolescents diagnosed with autism spectrum disorder (ASD). About sixty-eight percent of their sample population with autism spectrum disorder (ASD) displayed aggressive behavior towards their peers (Kanne & Mazurek, 2011). Conversely, about forty-nine percent of children and adolescents did not reveal any aggressive behavior. Kanne & Mazurek (2011) conducted their research with 1,380 adolescents between thirteen and seventeen who developed aggressive behaviors. In this study, males are more aggressive than females (Fitzpatrick, Srivorakiat, et al., 2016). However, gender has not been found to have a relationship with aggression in youth with autism spectrum disorder (ASD) (Fitzpatrick et al., 2016). Overall, the mission is to understand better how abnormal behavior causes a negative effect between family functioning, school, and social competence. (Simó-Pinatella et al., 2019).

Autism spectrum disorder (ASD) influences how individuals interact socially with their peers (Raulston et al., 2019). Adolescence who have autism experience difficulties with their learning, thinking, and problem-solving abilities (Raulston et al., 2019). Davis (2017) acknowledges how individuals with autism spectrum disorder (ASD) are educated to communicate and behave in various ways. Autistic individuals are taught to communicate effectively through American Sign Language (ASL), technology, reading, writing, and creating sounds (Raulston et al., 2019). Aggression has had a significant impact on adolescents with autism spectrum disorder (ASD). The second chapter will be addressing several strategies to reduce combative behaviors, which are applied behavior analysis (ABA), risk factors of autism spectrum disorder (ASD), teaching strategies, behavior strategies, triggers of aggression, outcomes of aggressive behaviors in adolescence, genetics, abuse, neglect, and quality of life in autism spectrum disorder (ASD). The purpose of this study is to identify the factors that are affiliated with aggressive behaviors (Raulston et al., 2019).

Applied Behavior Analysis (ABA)

Applied behavior analysis (ABA) teaches a person how to use several techniques to manage behavior problems in adolescence with autism spectrum disorder (ASD) (Slocum et al., 2014). Applied behavior analysis (ABA) is one of the most effective ways to teach a child with autism to improve their academics, speech, and decision-making skills (Slocum et al., 2014). In addition, however, behavior analysis is a valuable tool to educate and teach daily living skills to adolescence with autism spectrum disorder (ASD) (Slocum et al., 2014). The purpose of applied behavior analysis (ABA) is to increase appropriate behaviors like social skills, reading, communication, hygiene, and fine motor skills (Slocum et al., 2014).

There are many techniques for adolescence with autism to maintain positive behavior (Slocum et al., 2014). For example, applied behavior analysis (ABA) utilizes technology for youth with autism spectrum disorder (ASD) (Slocum et al., 2014). There are at least five ideas to create a change. These are touch screen tablets, computer applications, assistive communication devices, digital timers, and DVDs players are effective ways to reinforce positive behavior (Slocum et al., 2014). Technology is an alternative form for adolescence with autism to express themselves and improve their educational outcomes (Slocum et al., 2014). Besides, applied behavior analysis (ABA) will educate the child on effectively communicating their wants and needs (Kostewicz et al., 2016). It is essential to observe their behaviors and determine how to measure them with data (Kostewicz et al., 2016). Applied behavior analysis's objective is to (ABA) implement a change and produce a more significant impact on autism (Kostewicz et al., 2016).

Risk Factors of Aggression among Adolescents with ASD

Moreover, risk factors are associated with aggression among young adults and adolescents (Grinnell et al., 2019). This problematic abnormal behavior interferes with classroom learning and causes an individual with fewer opportunities for independent functioning and interpersonal relationships (Grinnell et al., 2019). It is also essential to recognize the impact of an autism diagnosis for parents because of their child's violent behavior (Grinnell et al., 2019). Therefore, social workers and care coordinators strive to support adolescents with autism to discuss peer interactions, educational goals, classroom placement, and aggressive behaviors (Grinnell et al., 2019).

Aggression can significantly impact someone's learning ability, and it is also unsafe for adults to handle aggressive behaviors (Sullivan et al., 2019). Parents begin to struggle with many problems when their child behaves aggressively (Sullivan et al., 2019). Additionally, aggression limits opportunities for the child to develop social relationships with others. For instance, if an individual with autism does not want to be near large crowds or loud noises, then the parent or caretaker should remove themselves from the situation to prevent the behavior from occurring (Sullivan et al., 2019). Sullivan et al. (2019) explain how it is crucial to understand the triggers of aggressive behaviors when they cannot communicate their thoughts and needs.

Teaching Strategies

Escorcia (2018) reveals how it is vital to meet the needs of individuals with autism who have experienced challenging behaviors. For example, the parent would have to tell their story or give a model to describe the situations they may find difficult or needs to help their child with autism spectrum disorder (ASD) (Escorcia, 2018). There are many additional resources in the school system to assist families who will need a support system: case managers, therapists, medical professionals, and some mental health providers (Escorcia, 2018). However, these team members will help address physical, mental, and learning concerns to create a supportive plan for challenging behaviors (Escorcia, 2018). The purpose of their involvement is to help people with autism grow, adapt, and empower families to focus on their strengths and challenges in life. Escorcia (2018) noted that families must build a team to develop specialized and individualized care for their loved ones.

Behavioral Strategies

Social skills can teach adolescents with autism spectrum disorder (ASD) some behavioral techniques to prevent them from having inappropriate outbursts (Escorcia, 2018). An adolescent with autism spectrum disorder (ASD) can learn how to react to social situations (Escorcia, 2018). There are modifying strategies to teach children to Stop-Observe-Deliberate-Act (SODA), created specifically for autism spectrum disorder (ASD) adolescents. Stop-Observe-Deliberate-Act (SODA) is a social learning strategy developed for adolescent participants (Escorcia, 2018). Furthermore, learning strategies can teach an adolescent to monitor their thinking and select effectively. The Stop-Observe-Deliberate-Act (SODA) steps will assist an adolescent with autism spectrum disorder (ASD) to improve their social interaction skills (Escorcia, 2018).

Triggers of Aggression

Aggression is characterized by physical or verbal behavior that could potentially cause harm to someone else (Fitzpatrick et al., 2016). Fitzpatrick et al. (2016) clarify how aggressive behaviors can be maladaptive or adaptive. Adaptive aggression is typically carried out to ensure the survival of an individual. (Escorcia, 2018). Maladaptive aggression is aggression that is unusually intense for its circumstances (Escorcia, 2018). Low I.Q., early language delays, low income, early maternal childbearing, and low parental education are linked to increased aggression risk (Kanne & Mazurek, 2011).

In normal development, aggressive behavior improves as children learn to regulate their emotions (Kaartinen et al., 2014). Autism does not develop normally; this is not always the case in children with an autism spectrum disorder (ASD). May et al. (2012) noted aggressive behavior is potentially higher in individuals with autism spectrum disorder (ASD). Individuals with autism spectrum disorder (ASD) have impairments in social interactions, lack of communication, repetitiveness, and behaviors that can be associated with intense aggression (Kaartinen et al., 2014). May et al. (2012) displayed data that the more severe the symptoms of autism are, the higher the risk will be for developing psychopathologies and problem behaviors like physical aggression.

Outcomes of Aggression with ASD

When combined with intellectual disabilities, individuals with autism spectrum disorder (ASD) are more likely to exhibit self-injurious and aggressive behaviors (Brentani et al., 2013). Brentani et al. (2013) mention how aggression is linked to several adverse outcomes for both the victim and the perpetrator. Adolescence with aggressive behaviors can be linked to crisis intervention, re-referrals, continuous readmission to residential facilities, use of psychotropic medications, and quality of life (Brentani et al., 2013). In other words, aggressive behaviors can lead to out-of-home placements for individuals with intellectual disabilities (Brentani et al., 2013).

A social worker must support individuals with developmental and intellectual disabilities, and it's essential to ensure autistic individuals can maintain good health by providing them medication (Maskey et al., 2013). Many participants who are autistic, therefore, struggle to be ial and functionally communicative. For many of these individuals, dication use could increase their independence and minimize their behaviors (Maskey et al., 2013). In addition, their inappropriate behaviors could lead the child not to become aggressive towards themselves and others (Maskey et al., 2013).

Additionally, there have been other medications that have been discontinued due to the side effects on the individual (Raulston et al., 2019). In some instances, some autistic individuals are required to be placed in a hospital or institutionalized setting to be sedated, restrained, or isolated from the family and caregivers (Raulston et al., 2019). For example, a 17-year-old autistic boy does not live with his family because of his behavioral problems. As a result, the boy has been placed in an institutionalized environment to treat his aggressive behaviors (Raulston et al., 2019). However, the caregiver has been working with the boy for at least ten years, and he has become an (AFL), which stands for alternative family living (Raulston et al., 2019). Assisted family living aims to provide a permanent and safe home for autistic participants (Raulston et al., 2019). Unfortunately, the parents could no longer support their child's needs, so instead, he was placed in assisted family living (AFL). The boy now lives with his long-time caretaker because of the lack of care from his biological parents (Raulston et al., 2019).

Genetics in Adolescence with ASD

Davis (2017) reveals how brain development has several factors, including gene mutations of autism. Navon et al. (2016) indicate how brain development is associated with autism spectrum disorder (ASD) genetics. While aggression is typical in individuals with autism spectrum disorder (ASD), no studies have examined its prevalence and the risk factors for its development (Hsiao, 2018). Hsiao (2018) clarifies how a person's genes can influence the outcome of certain traits 50% of the time. Research on gene-environment interaction has shown that genes are related to aggression (Kaartinen et al., 2014). Specifically, the monoamine oxidase gene is associated with an attack in individuals with autism (Kaartinen et al., 2014).

Abuse and Neglect in Adolescence with ASD

Furthermore, teenagers with autism spectrum disorder (ASD) are at a higher risk of abuse and neglect than children without disabilities (Regnault et al., 2018). Adolescents with autism who are exposed to having behavior issues may have experienced physical abuse. Parents and other adults must protect their children from mistreatment (Regnault et al., 2018). Misuse can cause a teenager to act out aggressively in public. However, parents must always know where the child is and ensure the child will be cared for in a place of harm and danger (Regnault et al., 2018). More importantly, caregivers and educators tend to be overwhelmed because of their child's abnormal behavior, and they do not know how to help their loved ones (Thurm & Swedo, 2012). Caregivers and educators should provide tools and techniques to help them understand why their child exhibits aggression towards others (Regnault et al., 2018).

Quality of Life in ASD

Aggressive behavior harms the quality of life for individuals with autism spectrum disorder (ASD) (Regnault et al., 2018). Therefore, challenging behaviors can also cause people to emotionally break down and burn out, including parents, teachers, and caregivers (Hodgetts et al., 2013). Therefore, it is essential to understand how aggression can interfere with their educational interventions, lack of empathy, social communication, and social interaction, amongst others (Hodgetts et al., 2013). In addition, adolescents with developmental disabilities develop aggressive behaviors as the strongest predictors of stress among parents (Raulston et al., 2019). Therefore, addressing aggressive behaviors will be highly beneficial to individuals with autism spectrum disorder (ASD) (Raulston et al., 2019).

The primary purpose of this study is to discover what factors contribute to aggression in adolescents with autism spectrum disorder (ASD) (Regnault et al., 2018). There is a high probability of aggressive behaviors in young adults with autism spectrum disorder (ASD) (Regnault et al., 2018). Also, negative factors can interfere with the child's success ability (Regnault et al., 2018). Aggressive behaviors in adolescents with autism spectrum disorder (ASD) can be challenging to diagnose when they cannot communicate their needs or concerns. This study incorporates how it is essential to help adolescents with autism learn new and effective methods to overcome aggressive behaviors (Regnault et al., 2018).

Chapter Three

Theoretical Framework

The purpose of chapter three is to discuss a theory that best explains aggressive behaviors in adolescents with autism spectrum disorder (ASD) (Mcleod, 2018). The selected approach is operant conditioning which is also identified as learning theory (Mcleod, 2018). Operant conditioning was chosen because it is a behavior learned through the classroom and environment (Mcleod, 2018). Operant conditioning is a skill performance that teaches students to learn through the consequences of behavior. Also, operant conditioning is a method to reward and punish inappropriate behaviors (Mcleod, 2018). This theory was selected because it teaches autistic individuals different skills on how to maintain good behavior. Overall, it is essential for adolescents with autism spectrum disorder (ASD) to learn creative ideas and reinforce positive behaviors (Mcleod, 2018).

Operant Conditioning

According to B. F. Skinner, operant theory stems from a learned standpoint (Mcleod, 2018). B. F. Skinner's operant conditioning model is implemented to teach, train, and manage abnormal behaviors (Mcleod, 2018). Operant conditioning is used to encourage good behavior than bad behavior. This theory can help improve communication, social interaction and decrease aggressive behaviors. In the research, behavior modification is one of the critical aspects of learning theory (Mcleod, 2018). Operant conditioning focuses on identifying behavior as positive reinforcement or negative reinforcement (Mcleod, 2018). This method of operant conditioning is used for autistic individuals to develop positive behaviors. The purpose of behavior modification is to reward students who maintain good behavior (Mcleod, 2018). For instance, each time the child cleans their room, the conditions for receiving their reward will change. This strategy can help people with autism and minimize their aggressive behaviors (Mcleod, 2018).

Positive reinforcement

B. F. Skinner acknowledges effective ways to teach an individual a learned behavior is positive reinforcement (Mcleod, 2018). Positive reinforcement motivates people to engage and increase positive behavior to receive an award (Mcleod, 2018). For example, an adolescent with autism spectrum disorder (ASD) will not have an outburst if they attend Ollies to purchase a book. However, they are more likely to perform this activity in the future (Mcleod, 2018). B. F. Skinner indicates how there is a variety of ideas to influence others to receive the results you want. Positive reinforcement is a unique way to motivate individuals with autism to develop skills, learn the rules, and encouraging them to do their best (Mcleod, 2018). The role of positive reinforcement is to establish new behaviors to maintain a productive lifestyle (Mcleod, 2018).

Negative reinforcement

B.F. Skinner developed negative reinforcement, which is also known as operant conditioning (Mcleod, 2018). Negative reinforcement is a behavior that removes or avoids an adverse outcome in exchange for an award. B. F. Skinner reveals how negative reinforcement is a technique to help children learn good patterns of behavior (Mcleod, 2018). For instance, some parents try to feed their children vegetables for dinner (Mcleod, 2018). However, the child does not like to eat the vegetables their parents are trying to give them. If the child sees any vegetables on their plate, then this will cause them to have a tantrum until they are taken off the plate (Mcleod, 2018). Instead, the child wanted to eat French fries, and their tantrums stopped (Mcleod, 2018). The purpose of negative reinforcement is when something is taken away because of something the child wanted (Mcleod, 2018).

Chapter Four

Addressing the Problem

Chapter Four will be discussing positive behavioral strategies in adolescence with autism spectrum disorder (ASD) (Kylliäinen et al., 2014). Kylliäinen et al. (2014) reveal how every student with autism spectrum disorder (ASD) is unique, with different strengths and needs. There are strategies to improve social and academic abilities for students diagnosed with autism. Also, Kylliäinen et al. (2014) explain how educational classrooms are made up of students with autism, and it is the teacher's goal to ensure their needs are met (Kylliäinen et al., 2014). Teachers should provide equal education for students diagnosed with autism. However, the school system should maintain to meet the necessities of several students diagnosed with autism spectrum disorder (ASD). The reasoning for this strategic plan is to create a caring and 4rcollaborative learning environments for all autistic students (Kylliäinen et al., 2014).

Some strategies can minimize abnormal behaviors and promote positive outcomes to meet the needs of adolescence with autism (Regnault et al., 2018). All adolescents with autism spectrum disorder (ASD) are different, and it is essential to try different strategies to create a change. The study will be a quantitative approach. There will be at least ten questions for the participants who have experienced aggressive behaviors in autism (Regnault et al., 2018). The student will attend at least two public schools who have aggressive behaviors in their classrooms. A survey design will be chosen to investigate the factors in adolescence with autism spectrum disorder (ASD) (Regnault et al., 2018).

Positive reinforcement is a proactive strategy for dealing with adolescent problem behaviors with autism spectrum disorder (ASD) (Regnault et al., 2018). Positive reinforcement would be an effective way for staff members and teachers to manage abnormal behaviors. The participants will reward the child with special privileges to decrease their adverse outcomes (Regnault et al., 2018). For instance, the staff will give the student a cookie if they are well behaved in the classroom. In addition, the team will bribe the student to reduce negative behaviors. However, the survey will be face-to-face for the participants to complete in hand (Regnault et al., 2018). The survey focus will be positive reinforcement so staff members can learn the tools and techniques to minimize behaviors. The questionnaire will be multiple-choice, and it will provide practice questions to maintain positive behaviors. Most of those questions will consist of demographics and positive reinforcement strategies to decrease behaviors (Regnault et al., 2018). Also, the students will provide fifteen surveys for each of those schools to complete. The survey tool will be based on implementing a change and asking the community to acknowledge their suggestions on reducing abnormal behaviors (Regnault et al., 2018).

The goal would be to count how many individuals with autism exhibit aggressive behaviors in the classroom setting (Regnault et al., 2018). The participants conducting this research have experience interacting with individuals who have autism. This research will explore the behaviors of many individuals with temper tantrums (Regnault et al., 2018). All the participants of this study will receive information about the practical strategies of positive reinforcement and how it manages aggressive behaviors before the survey is completed (Regnault et al., 2018).

Additionally, the focal point of this research proposal is to analyze the factors for adolescents with autism who have behavioral problems (Kostewicz et al., 2016). The abnormal behaviors need to be addressed, and it is essential to display how serious it is to increase awareness for people with autism spectrum disorder (ASD) (Kostewicz et al., 2016). Not to mention how important it is to support individuals with autism and their families with resources, online tools, and information for people who are disabled (Kostewicz et al., 2016). Therefore, the behavioral issues of adolescents with autism spectrum disorder (ASD) will be displayed in a graph. This will explain whether there has been significant growth for aggressive students (Kostewicz et al., 2016).

Chapter Five

Conclusion

Autism spectrum disorder (ASD) is a significant public health issue in our society (Hanley et al., 2014). It is challenging for adolescence with autism spectrum disorder (ASD) to interact with people because of their behavioral problems (Hanley et al., 2014). Adolescents with autism spectrum disorder (ASD) tend to struggle with isolation, anxiety, tantrums, and emotional reactions (Hanley et al., 2014). However, adolescence with autism spectrum disorder (ASD) behavioral and social problems should be minimized to meet their educational needs (Hanley et al., 2014). It is essential for adolescents with autism spectrum disorder (ASD) to learn how to communicate their needs and participate in society. Chapter five will discuss how families should have access to education and treatment opportunities to reach their fullest potential (Hanley et al., 2014).

Social Work Implication

This research proposal implies how social workers should provide parents with community resources and educational goal planning to prevent aggressive behaviors (Hanley et al., 2014). A social worker ensures the students are provided with all the needed support to reduce aggressive behaviors (Hanley et al., 2014). Social workers are often involved in the evaluation of students' behavior plans (Hanley et al., 2014). Also, a social worker's role is to advocate to support people with intellectual and developmental disabilities and create a fundamental change in their lives (Hanley et al., 2014). To help adolescents with autism could include support groups, family therapy, and discussions at home and school interventions about community resources available (Hanley et al., 2014). Families can find support groups in several ways: schools, agencies, doctors, and social networking. Support groups help families, friends, and peers understand how autism spectrum disorder (ASD) affects their quality of life (Hanley et al., 2014).

On the other hand, students diagnosed with autism spectrum disorder (ASD) educational goals will be assessed (Hodgetts et al.,2013). All students who receive specialized services in an academic setting have an individualized Educational Plan (IEP) that distinguishes their personalized goals (Hodgetts et al.,2013). The purpose of an individualized Educational Plan (IEP) is designed for parents and teachers to advocate for their child's educational goals. In addition, the individualized Educational Plan (IEP) determines the child's placement, needs, and the school district's ability to provide an environment conducive to learning (Hodgetts et al.,2013).

There are many valuable resources for parents struggling with behavior issues (Hodgetts et al.,2013). There are tools and techniques to help them understand why their children show aggression towards others (Hodgetts et al.,2013). Aggressive behavior harms the quality of life for individuals with autism spectrum disorder (ASD). Therefore, aggressive behaviors can cause people to emotionally break down, including parents, teachers, and caregivers (Hodgetts et al., 2013). Also, it is vital to understand how aggression can interfere with their educational interventions, lack of empathy, social communication, and social interaction, amongst others (Hodgetts et al.,2013). Therefore, the teachers, parents, and caregivers must work with the students to increase positive behaviors with autism spectrum disorder (ASD). This way, the behaviors, and aggressiveness could reduce the frequency of the challenging behavioral issues (Hodgetts et al., 2013).

What is Theoretical Orientation?

The concept of theoretical orientation is for the professional to find a productive method to better serve their client in need. Theoretical orientation is an effective way to become a helpful professional to integrate your learning and practice. To become a therapist, it is essential to understand the different theories of how someone's issue develops and how to solve the problem. Every client is different and has theories depending on the client's needs. It is crucial to choose an effective tool that would be a great fit for the client (Healy, 2014).

As social workers grow and adapt in their profession; it would be very beneficial for them to continue learning more about their theory-based approach (Healy, 2014). In the social work profession, the more you work with clients you can determine what does your toolbox has to offer. The goal is to further assist our clients from the pain, suffering, and more towards fulfillment (Cascio et al., 2016). Theories of counseling will continue to have a positive outcome in their lives (Healy, 2014). I believe learning about the different types of theoretical orientation frameworks will determine the most effective way to move forward to improve the client's well-being. The idea of theoretical orientation tends to have a unique sense of style and self-discovery (Healy, 2014).

Experience of Theoretical Orientation

My theoretical orientation would be the strengths-based approach in the field of social work. The strengths-based approach focuses on positivity rather than negativity. In my field, working with individuals with Intellectual and Developmental disabilities can develop more positive attributes and affect change within themselves. I learned special needs individuals are very different and unique in their artistic way. They all have their own story and come from entirely different backgrounds. Autistic individuals are also sensitive and can sense the tension of a person who may be in a bad mood. People with special needs are very intelligent, they can sense your negativity, verbal, non-verbal expression, facial expressions, and body language (Cascio et al, 2016). If so, they will become agitated and develop abnormal behavior because of another individual's negativity. Throughout my life, I learned you leave your problems at home, put a smile on your face, and conduct a positive mindset to better serve your clients.

Discourses shaped Theoretical Orientation

As a leader, I have learned working with individuals on the autism spectrum needs should be always met. We must implement strategic goal planning and interact with the family, teachers, and other professionals to conduct more Individualized Education Programs (IEP). With this, individuals with autism will have the opportunity to focus more on their strength's perspectives (Macmillan, 2021). The objective of the Individualized Education Program (IEP) is for families to determine their child's fundamental level of learning to work within a positive environment (Macmillan, 2021). The strengths-based approach will decrease their level of uncertainty and abnormal behaviors. The strengths perspective theoretical approach will highlight their positive areas of interest to increase their level of functioning. Another is mental health can affect their social interactions and learn within the classroom environment (Macmillan, 2021).

Integrated new Perspectives

Mental health can negatively prevent individuals with autism from gaining knowledge and new skills (Macmillan, 2021). Mental health interventions support the needs of each child to help their level of anxiety (Macmillan et al, 2021). A helpful strategy would be to attempt to collaborate, advocate, and plan to put unique ideas into place for their success (Duggal et al., 2020). As professionals, it is vital that we help individuals with autism with their needs, rights, aspirations, self-esteem, self-confidence, build relationships, and communication skills

(Carter et al., 2020). Children of autism want to be happy, supported, loved, and understood because they can sense their understanding of learning (Carter et al., 2020). As social workers, we are the alternative voice for these creative individuals and our objective is to increase their long-term positive effects (Carter et al., 2020).

Autistic individuals have the capacities, courage, character, resourcefulness, and the possibilities to overcome their challenges (McConachie et al., 2015). All these assets that were listed will guide them towards the right path to reach their ambitions (Duggal et al., 2020). From a strength standpoint, I believe focusing on the individuals' strengths will help participants achieve specific desired outcomes to overcome their future aspirations. The strengths perspective is a very powerful technique that aligns people with autism the inner and outer resources to improve the quality of their life (McConachie et al., 2015).

Diversity and Inclusion

To better enhance our ability to serve special needs it is vital to exercise diversity in a different light (Beck, 2018). From the social workers' perspective, we strive to advocate and speak on their behalf to maintain healthy relationships. Social workers must motivate people with disabilities towards expanding their knowledge and self-improvement (Beck, 2018). The solution-based theory will also fall into place once the social worker receives the adequate resources to increase their activity of daily living (McConachie et al., 2015). While working in the special need's profession, I learned how to treat every individual equally no matter the circumstances. In addition, I was taught to never mistreat people because you would want someone to treat you with the same equality, dignity, and respect. Additionally, all individuals with autism are entitled to receive all the resources and equal opportunities for their success (Duggal et al., 2020). The role is to strengthen their natural abilities to create positive and productive outcomes (McConachie et al., 2015).

Leadership Style

I am hopeful as a therapist, I will be able to value my client's empowerment, so the family can help their child to determine themselves. As a leader, it is important to meet the clients' basic needs for recognition, equal treatment, and appreciation which is crucial in a therapeutic relationship (McConachie et al., 2015). Leadership is about setting an example to motivate people to grow and elevate to a higher level of achievement (McConachie et al., 2015). Therefore. I chose to discuss the strengths perspective because a leader helps other change, develop, and succeed. I am willing to inspire autistic individuals to concentrate on their strengths to find better alternatives.

I think it is necessary to recognize your strengths to work towards achieving goals. As we go through life, we must learn who we are, so we can identify how to adapt, and grow from our strengths. Children on the autism spectrum will need all the guidance, love encouragement, and support to identify their level of independence. Individuals with special needs have the capabilities to underline their strengths and seek for alternatives to implement a change. The solution-based theory will further along guide children of autism to find positive interests in things that are enjoyable to them. A social worker should be a leader who brainstorms ideal outcomes so individuals with autism can reach their fullest potential.

Social Change

Social change focuses on human interactions and the way people tend to react towards one another (Christopher & Shakila, 2015). When you are open to adapt to change then will have more opportunities and responsibilities. In special education, it is vital to embrace new experiences and new consequences. Individuals with special needs began to learn and grow as a person to figure out a better path in their lifetime. In other words, social change is good in a positive way because it makes a positive difference in our society. It is vital to understand the child's needs to improve their quality of life (Christopher & Shakila, 2015). Many children with autism may be experiencing abuse, neglect, mental health, dysfunctional households, and other issues in the world. So, we must consider all these factors to have a more idea of what they are feeling (Christopher & Shakila, 2015). That is why it is essential to brainstorm innovative methods and ideas to meet the needs of autistic children. Meanwhile, the concept of social innovation is a way to design strategic ideas for a pathway of change (Christopher & Shakila, 2015). As a social worker, it is important to acknowledge that the lack of social skills is a learned behavior through other interactions. In the social work profession, we need to continue to raise awareness so children can learn to interact socially (Christopher & Shakila, 2015).

Mindfulness of ASD

Ethical leadership implements an environment where the goals and values of people working in an organization. We must remember that everyone is an individual, and we must assess their perspectives with shared values. With ethical leadership it is important to demonstrate your character and values to others. To display ethical leadership it is essential to have the background knowledge on how to handle or what to do if there is a situation.

Ethical leadership focuses on the needs and rights. It is vital to treat every individual equally as a human being. I believe someone who is ethical is honest, straightforward, and holding everyone to the same standards. Mindfulness is the state of observing one's thoughts and feelings without judging. Mindfulness is about doing the right thing to help you understand yourself better and improve quality of life. Ethical leaders and mindfulness both intersect because any person in a leadership position who wants to continue in their leadership role would be wise to practice their mindfulness.

A successful leader is one who is cognizant of their team's emotional wellbeing as well as their physical. Moreover, we must be mindful of others because it is important to show respect and embrace kindness to become a better person. That is why I am a advocate of mindfulness because we must value our differences which is a way of being in life. Working with individuals of special needs have empowered me to strengthen my social and emotional intelligence. Assisting individuals on the autism spectrum was a way for me learn how to love myself even more. I am grateful to be in the position to be of service to others who needs guidance throughout their lives.

Mindfulness shapes people with autism into better human beings that gives them a sense of meaning to view the world in a peaceful place.

Community Advocate

According to Izquierdo (2012) "We can achieve many goals within its time frame". To be a great leader, it is vital to communicate with our mentors, peers, and speak up, and fight for what we believe is right (Izquierdo, 2012). I can say that I have several experiences at the macro-level of social work. One experience I enjoyed was being a Guardian ad Litem. I used to be a Guardian ad Litem for individuals with autism before I went back to graduate school. In 2017, I had to resign as a Guardian ad Litem because my objective was to focus on my studies, internship, commuting to class, and the workload, so, therefore, I had no time to continue this wonderful experience of working with individuals in need. I remember I was appointed a case to prove to the judge my right was in the best interest of the children. I had two twin boys and at the time they were one year old. They were very sweet, loving, gentle, adorable, and both were very playful, even though one cried more than the other.

The mother was abusing drugs, had no car, no home, was unemployed, and had a lack of support system. The father had decent employment, but he was not attending court and not answering phone calls. The father had a lack of interest to be a part of his children's lives. The mother had arrangements to see her children weekly for two hours under supervision. However, the twins moved from foster home to the next. Their first foster home was accused of physical abuse. So, the boys had to get adjusted to a new environment which was very difficult for them. They both were in daycare; I remember I visited them to see how the twins adapted to a new atmosphere. They seemed to be very happy and enjoyed playing with the other babies. The day program was providing me with updates on how the boys had been progressing. I was pleased to observe them interact with people of disabilities to increase their socialization skills.

Izquierdo (2012) mentions how a leader needs to have good communication skills to deliver the message. Advocates develop a strategic plan and a different approach for every issue (Izquierdo, 2012). This is the reason why I spent my entire time out in the field collaborating with social workers, teachers, foster parents, and other medical professionals. As an advocate, my role was to attend home visits and doctor's appointments to look for anything suspicious that could affect their wellbeing. My goal was to speak for the children to ensure they were in a safe, secure, and productive household. I also kept in contact with the social worker, she was very informative about the circumstances of the children's lives. The social worker also shared confidential information, so I could pitch in and help locate community resources for the sake of the children (Izquierdo, 2012). Afterward, I learned so much being a leader within the community, I began to learn more about the twins individually. As time passed, I learned more about their strengths and weakness. One twin was fully developing than the other. One was walking while the other was crawling, or one was eating food rather than baby food.

Overall, being a leader had educated me a lot about my strengths and weakness. I leaned in the macro-level of social work, it is essential to focus more on your strengths to increase positivity and self-confidence. I began to develop a positive mindset then everything had fallen into place, I can say I did make mistakes. But I learned to asked questions, listen, stay focused, and you will improve along the way. It was an incredible journey being a Guardian ad Litem, and I was delighted to have the opportunity to be an advocate.

My Own Boss

Ever since I was a little girl, I have always dreamed of becoming an entrepreneur. I loved the feeling of becoming a leader. Leadership has inspired me to achieve a certain goal through direction and motivation. I am passionate to give back to the community by helping vulnerable individuals who were in need. I have always been in the eyes of what my surroundings wanted me to accomplish in life. Now, as I have grown up, I realized that now it is my time to shine and work on my path towards making my own decisions. We all have a dream to become our own boss. We all want to follow our own set of rules in our lifetime. Therefore, we cannot let anything hold us back from achieving our goals.

I learned in life if you want something then go for it. Do not stop! Do not wait! Do not let anyone or anything prevent you from growing in any other aspects of life. Therefore I have a dream to continue to focus on creating an empire and advocating for individuals with disabilities because their opportunities are ignored in our society. I want to give individuals with special needs a chance to freedom, growth, happiness, independently, and a fulfilling life. We all have talents, abilities, and limits to improve their confidence and quality of life.

Note: If you want to be your own boss, please be adventurously creative towards developing a new empire. We must not settle for less, many of us do not realize we can implement anything were passionate about. So I would advise you to please think of something that brings you joy and happiness. Write down at least five things your passionate about then you will begin to bring your own vision to life.

Jewell's of Autism L.L.C.

1. **Background and**

   a. **Company history**
   Jewell's of autism will provide special education services to meet the needs of students with disabilities. Special education will offer unique resources to fulfill the students' performance in learning. The day program will provide individualized instruction, smaller classroom settings, and highly trained professionals to educate the students academically and behaviorally.

   b. **What we do**
   Jewell's of autism will only provide day program services from 8 am to 5 pm. The adult day program will ensure to provide care for elderly people and other adults who are 18 and over. We will require personal care services, protective supervision, and assistance in the activities of daily living. There will be planned activities which will include art, music, dancing, discussion, support groups, and technology. In addition, the adult day program will assist students with teaching, coaching, self-advocacy, and community integration to enrich their wellbeing.

2. Strategy & Vision

a. Vision statement
Our vision for Jewell's of autism will implement a productive learning organization to equally educate students with special needs. There will be opportunities for growth of success, so every student has unique individual needs. We will continue to educate our leaders who can reach their long-term goals in the school setting and community.

b. Mission statement
Our mission would be to cultivate a safe and secure environment to increase the lifelong effects for students with Intellectual and Developmental disabilities. We will strive for excellence and provide our clients the best possible service through specialized care, dignity, and acceptance.

c. Values
Jewell's of autism will treat all our people equally with dignity, respect, and courtesy. We will always collaborate and work together as a team no matter the circumstances. We will always remain humble, strong, positive, honest, and fair in all our actions. We will hold ourselves accountable for our actions, continue to advocate, and do the right thing to celebrate the success of clients' accomplishments. We are in it to win it!

d. Business goals & objectives
Jewell's of autism's goal is to ensure all our client's basic needs and services are met within their activity of daily living. We will enhance their sensory skills, fine motor, personal interactions, social communications, and gross motor skills to empower students to expand their learning capabilities.

e. **Growth strategy**

Jewell's of autism is willing to collaborate and partner with several organizations and communities to allocate the necessary resources to keep the business successful long-term. We will continue to raise the awareness of autism through flyers, brochures, blogs, social networking, and other productive ways to promote the business effectively.

3. Finances & Services

a. **Finances**

Jewell's of Autism will have a business account set up to ensure our company is flowing accordingly as planned. The adult day program will document all our assists, losses, gains, etc. to ensure we are within our budget. More importantly, Jewell's of Autism will ensure everyone is aware of their pay rate, vacation, sick leave, maternity leave, time off, bonuses, holiday pay, overtime, paid time off, and other incentives that will be provided to our staff.

b. **Services**

Jewell's of Autism will provide care, companionship, assistance, and supervision during the day. Jewell's of Autism will serve our student's recreation, social activities, varying levels of medical services, and transportation. Adult day services are a resource for our staff and clients to determine how the adult day program will benefit their health and well-being. Jewells of Autism will encourage one another to spend time with others to improve daily living skills. Adult day service will give people the opportunity to feel safe, secured, and comfortable in a new environment.

c. **Business competitiveness**

Jewell's of Autism will be in a safe and spacious environment for all our customers. The day program will ensure there is available parking space for our clients. The program will be in our atmosphere to provide family support and services. Jewell's of Autism will be aware of other day program services that will be provided to our customers, parents, and staff. The day program will assure our staff and clients will explore the facility to ensure this is the right fit to meet their basic needs. It is our responsibility the program will respect their decision no matter the circumstances. Adult day program provides a productive environment for all who we serve.

4. Management & Ownership

a. Owner/Director: Sydney McGee will be responsible to oversee the daily operations of the facility, funds, and budgets to maintain an effective program. The director will organize and lead staff meetings and may attend clinical, individual support plan, which is identified as ISP meetings. The program director will ensure the workers and clients are in a safe and secure environment. The director will manage to educate staff, implement a curriculum in coordination with workers, communicate with parents to strengthen the program's reputation.

b. Program Director: N/A will be responsible for managing the clients and staff within the day program service. The program director will ensure that the program is in line with the companies' objectives. They will oversee callouts, training, monitor the progress on goals, provide staff within the day program. The director of the program will coordinate the daily activities and local community outings for staff and clients. They will be required to attend clinical and individual support plans (ISP). They will step in, and cover shifts if there is no staff available. Also, the program director will ensure integrity is put into place to oversee if the objectives of the program are met.

c. Clinical Supervisor: Tia Black will oversee healthcare workers and clients daily. The clinical supervisor will lead, coach, and mentor to make sure staff meet the standards of all applicable laws and regulations. The clinical supervisor will maintain clinical records, inventory, clinic equipment, and clinic reports. They will create and manage schedules to ensure the staff is clocking in and out their time correctly. They will have direct contact with the family to report any questions or concerns, and callouts regarding the day program services. The clinical supervisor will review, become a future hiring manager, manage budget, perform reviews, and assess treatment plans to evaluate the level of patient care.

"Anything Is possible! If I can do it, so can you!"

Note: *Anything is possible if you just believe in yourself. Not everything is not possible. Whatever a mind an conceive and believe, the mind can achieve. I believe we as humans can achieve anything because we are the ones who can accomplish them. We are the ones who can make just hope for a better result in a positive manner. Please follow your passion, strength, and inner peace to accomplish anything.*

Reference

Beck, S. L., (2018). Developing and writing a diversity statement. Vanderbilt University Center for Teaching. https://cft.vanderbilt.edu/developing-and-writing-a-diversity-statement**es**

Brentani, Helena, Paula, Cristiane Silvestre de, Bordini, Daniela, Rolim, Deborah, Sato, Fabio, Portolese, Joana, Pacifico, Maria Clara, & McCracken, James T. (2013). Autism spectrum disorders: an overview of diagnosis and treatment. *Brazilian Journal of Psychiatry, 35*(Suppl. 1), S62-S72. https://dx.doi.org/10.1590/1516-4446-2013-S104.

Buon, M., Dupoux, E., Jacob, P., Chaste, P., Leboyer, M., & Zalla, T. (2013). The role of causal and intentional judgments in moral reasoning in individuals with high functioning autism. *Journal of Autism and Developmental Disorders, 43*(2), 458-70.

Cascio CJ, Woynaroski T, Baranek GT, Wallace MT. (2016). Toward an interdisciplinary approach to understanding sensory function in autism spectrum disorder. Autism Res. 20;9(9):920-5. doi: 10.1002/aur.1612. Epub 2016 Apr 19. PMID: 27090878. PMCID: PMC5564205.

Carter EW, Carlton ME, Travers HE. (2020). Seeing strengths: young adults and them siblings with autism or intellectual disability. J Appl Res Intellect Disable. 2020 May;33(3):574-583. doi: 10.1111/jar.12701. PMID: 31919930; PMCID: PMC7160005

Centers for Disease Control and Prevention. (2013). National Health Interview Survey. Retrieved from http://www.cdc.gov/asthma /nis/2013/table1-1.htm.

Christopher, S.& Shakila, C. (2015). Social Skills in Children with Autism. 10.13140/RG.2.2.20772.78724.

Duggal, C., Dua, B., Chokhani, R., & Sengupta, K. (2020). What works and how: Adult learner perspectives on an autism intervention training program in India. Autism, 24(1), 246–257. https://doi.org/10.1177/1362361319856955

Escorcia, A. V. (2018). *Understanding aggressive behavior in children with autism spectrum disorder* (Order No. 13419132). Available from ProQuest Central; ProQuest Dissertations & Theses Global. (2269386781). http://nclive.org.ezproxy.nccu.edu/cgi-bin/nclsm?url=http://search.proquest.com.ezproxy.nccu.edu/docview/2269386781?accountid=12713

Fitzpatrick, S. E., Srivorakiat, L., Wink, L. K., Pedapati, E. V., & Erickson, C. A. (2016). Aggression in autism spectrum disorder: presentation and treatment options. *Neuropsychiatric disease and treatment, 12*, 1525–1538.

Grinnell, R. M., Williams, M., & Unrau, Y. A. (2019). Research methods for social workers: An introduction. Copyright 2019.: Pair Bond Publications.

Hanley, G. P., Jin, C. S., Vanselow, N. R., & Hanratty, L. A. (2014). Producing meaningful improvements in the problem behavior of children with autism via synthesized analysis and treatments. 47(1),16-36.

Hodgetts, S., Nicholas, D., & Zwaigenbaum, L. (2013). Home Sweet Home? Families' Experiences with Aggression in Children with Autism Spectrum Disorders. *Focus on Autism and Other Developmental Disabilities, 28*(3), 166–174. https://doi.org/10.1177/1088357612472932

Healy, K. (2014). *Social work theories in context: Creating frameworks for practice* (2nd ed.). Red Globe Press.

Hsiao, Y. (2018). Parental stress in families of children with disabilities. *Intervention in School and Clinic, 53*(4), 201-205. Retrieved from http://nclive.org.ezproxy.nccu.edu/cgi-bin/nclsm?url=http://search.proquest.com.ezproxy.nccu.edu/docview/2023999886?accountid=1713

Kaartinen, M., Puura, K., Helminen, M., Salmelin, R., Pelkonen, E., & Juujärvi, P. (2014). Reactive aggression among children with and without autism spectrum disorder. *Journal of Autism and Developmental Disorders, 44*(10), 2383-91.

Kanne, S. M., & Mazurek, M. O. (2011). Aggression in children and adolescents with ASD: Prevalence and risk factors. *Journal of Autism and Developmental Disorders, 41*(7), 926-37.

Kylliäinen, A., Jones, E.J.H., Gomot, M. (2014). Practical Guidelines for Studying Young Children with Autism Spectrum Disorder in Psychophysiological Experiments. *Rev J Autism Dev Disorder* **1**, 373–386.

Kostewicz, D. E., King, S. A., Datchuk, S. M., Brennan, K. M., & Casey, S. D. (2016). Data collection and measurement assessment in behavioral research: 1958–2013. Behavior analysis: Research and Practice, 16(1), 19-33.

Macmillan, C.M., Pecora, L.A., Ridgway, K. et al. (2021). An Evaluation of Education-Based Interventions for Students with Autism Spectrum Disorders Without Intellectual Disability: a Systematic Review. https://doi.org/10.1007/s40489-021-00289-0

McConachie H, Parr JR, Glod M, Hanratty J, Livingstone N, Oono IP, Robalino S, Baird G, Beresford B, Charman T, Garland D, Green J, Gringras P, Jones G, Law J, Le Couteur AS, Macdonald G, McColl EM, Morris C, Rodgers J, Simonoff E, Terwee CB, Williams K. (2015). systematic review of tools to measure outcomes for young children with autism spectrum disorder. Health Technol Assess.;19(41):1-506. doi: 10.3310/hta19410. PMID: 26065374; PMCID: PMC4781156.

Maskey, M., Warnell, F., Parr, J. R., Le Couteur, A., & McConachie, H. (2013). Emotional and behavioral problems in children with an autism spectrum disorder. *Journal of Autism and Developmental Disorders, 43*(4), 851-9.

May, M. E., Brandt, R. C., & Bohannan, J. K. (2012). Moderating Effects of Autism on Parent Views of Genetic Screening for Aggression. *Intellectual and Developmental Disabilities, 50*(5), 415-425.

Navon, D., & Eyal, G. (2016). Looping genomes: Diagnostic change and the genetic makeup of the autism population. *The American Journal of Sociology, 121*(5), 1416.

Niditch, L. A., Varela, R. E., Kamps, J. L., & Hill, T. (2012). Exploring the association between cognitive functioning and anxiety in children with autism spectrum disorders: The role of social understanding and aggression. *Journal of Clinical Child and Adolescent Psychology, 41*(2), 127.

Raulston, T. J., Hieneman, M., Caraway, N., Pennefather, J., & Bhana, N. (2019). Enablers of behavioral parent training for families of children with an autism spectrum disorder. *Journal of Child and Family Studies, 28*(3), 693-703. doi:http://dx.doi.org.ezproxy.nccu.edu/10.1007/s10826-018-1295-x

Regnault, A., Willgoss, T., Barbic, S. (2018). International Society for Quality of Life Research (ISOQOL) Mixed Methods Special Interest Group (SIG). Towards the use of mixed methods inquiry as best practice in health outcomes research. Journal of patient-reported outcomes, 2(1), 19. 10.1186/s41687-018-0043-8

Simó-Pinatella, D., Mumbardó-Adam, C., Alomar-Kurz, E., Sugai, G., & Simonsen, B. (2019).

Prevalence of challenging behaviors exhibited by children with disabilities: Mapping the literature. *Journal of Behavioral Education, 28*(3), 323-343. :http://dx.doi.org.ezproxy.nccu.edu/10.1007/s10864-019-09326-9

Slocum, T. A., Detrich, R., Wilczynski, S. M., Spencer, T. D., Lewis, T., & Wolfe, K. (2014). The Evidence-Based Practice of Applied Behavior Analysis. *The Behavior Analyst, 37*(1), 41–56. https://doi.org/10.1007/s40614-014-0005-2

Sullivan, M.O., Gallagher, L. & Heron, E.A. (2019). Gaining Insights into Aggressive Behavior in Autism Spectrum Disorder Using Latent Profile Analysis. *J Autism Dev Disorder* **49,** 4209–4218 (2019). https://doi.org/10.1007/s10803-019-04129-3

Thurm, A., & Swedo, S. E. (2012). The importance of autism research. Dialogues in clinical neuroscience, 14(3), 219–222